Heart Disease

Treating Heart Disease
Preventing Heart Disease

By Ace McCloud
Copyright © 2014

Disclaimer

The information provided in this book is designed to provide helpful information on the subjects discussed. This book is not meant to be used, nor should it be used, to diagnose or treat any medical condition. For diagnosis or treatment of any medical problem, consult your own physician. The publisher and author are not responsible for any specific health or allergy needs that may require medical supervision and are not liable for any damages or negative consequences from any treatment, action, application or preparation, to any person reading or following the information in this book. Any references included are provided for informational purposes only. Readers should be aware that any websites or links listed in this book may change.

Table of Contents

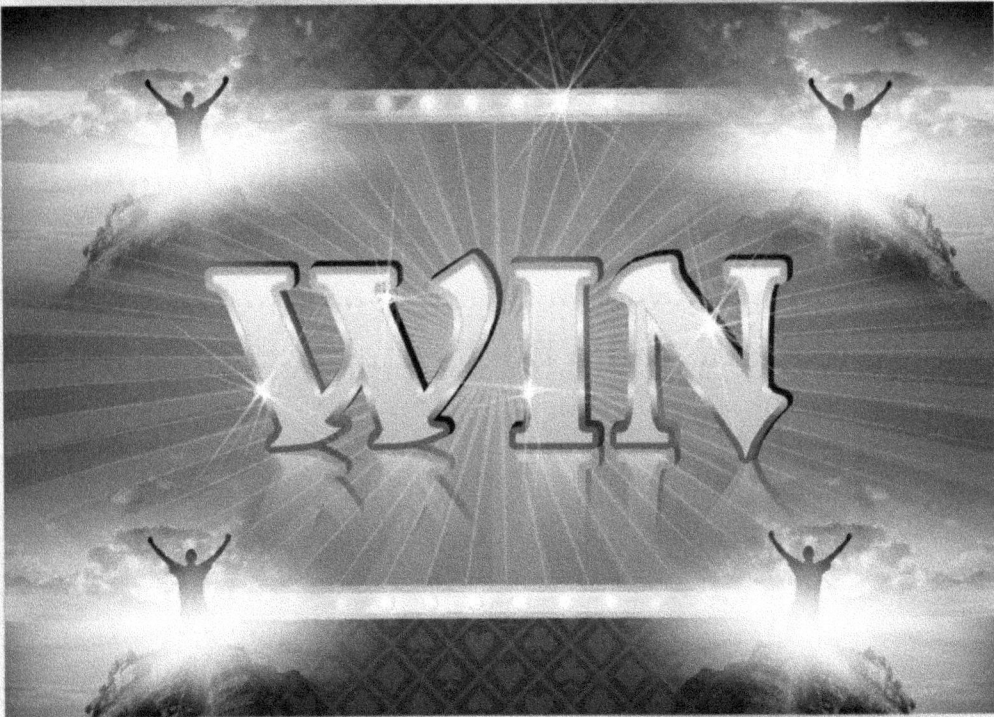

DEDICATED TO THOSE WHO ARE PLAYING THE GAME OF LIFE TO WIN

KEEP ON PUSHING AND NEVER GIVE UP!

Ace McCloud

Be sure to check out my website for all my Books and Audio books.

www.AcesEbooks.com

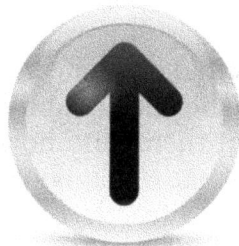

Introduction

I want to thank you and congratulate you for buying the book, "Heart Disease Cure: How To Treat Heart Disease, How To Prevent Heart Disease, All Natural Remedies, Medical Breakthroughs, And Proper Diet And Exercise For Heart Disease."

This book contains proven steps and strategies on how to handle different heart problems. Here you'll find the basics of different heart diseases, how conventional medicine helps treat them, and how natural approaches are equally effective in handling these problems. This book is aimed at encouraging you to take simple steps and make small lifestyle changes to boost your heart health. You'll discover everything from the best tips and tricks for boosting your heart health to natural foods and therapies that'll keep your heart happy and get you buzzing with health and joy!

Looking for that inspirational pat-on-the back to rev up your heart health? This book covers just that, and more. Basically, it's all you need to get started on a healthy journey that you'll actually enjoy, and notice great improvements in not just your heart health, but your overall well being too! So what are you waiting for? Get started on a whole new journey towards better health.

Remember that this book is NOT a replacement for professional medical advice. It is recommended that you visit a healthcare professional to seek advice regarding your heart health and to see how you can use the different parts of this book to help you make better choices in improving your heart health.

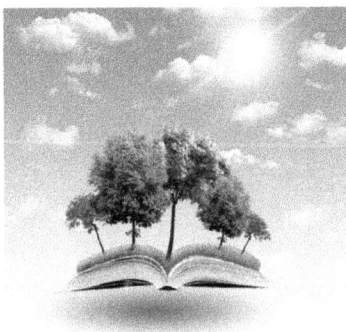

Chapter 1: Understanding the Basics

Heart disease is the most potentially life-threatening disease, and claims millions of lives worldwide every year. The past few decades has shown a steep rise in the number of people getting affected by this condition, which is even scarier.
While lifestyle and diet play an important role in determining the occurrence of heart diseases, certain genetic and hereditary factors have their own special place when it comes to increasing the risk of heart problems.

If you have a family history of heart disease, or already suffer from a cardiovascular condition, this book is for you. Here you'll understand the basics of your health condition, learn about how conventional medicines and drugs can help you manage it, and finally discover simple and natural approaches to dealing with the problem. So let's get started and understand what heart disease is all about.

Basically, heart disease, in general, refers to a group of disorders that affect the heart, and in turn, different organ systems of the body. While some heart diseases are very closely and directly linked to lifestyle choices and diet, a lot of heart diseases arise as a result of certain infections or genetic factors that are uncontrollable.

It is estimated that almost 1 out of every 3 Americans die of heart disease. Thankfully, due to public awareness, the death rate associated with heart disease is now decreasing.

Here are some of the most common heart diseases:

Coronary artery disease: Coronary artery disease is one of the most common heart diseases. It is basically a blockage in the coronary artery- which is responsible for supplying the blood to the heart. This blockage may result in a reduced supply of blood, which saps the heart muscles of the vital oxygen they require.

Coronary artery disease is believed to stem from atherosclerosis- a condition where the arteries of the heart get hardened, and do not allow blood to pass through them with ease. Coronary artery disease is linked to causing many other different heart diseases, including heart attack, angina (chest pain) and even sudden death. A sedentary lifestyle with poor eating habits, smoking, stress and genetic factors are all believed to be linked to this disease.

Arrhythmias: Arrhythmias is basically an abnormal beating pattern of the heart- it has a number of potential causes and is often a consequence of some other heart problems.

Heart failure: Contrary to what the term suggests, heart failure does not imply that the heart has stopped working; infact, it means that the heart is incapable of pumping out the amount of blood that's ideally required by the body. This disease is usually caused due to several other health conditions including thyroid disease, cardiomyopathy, high blood pressure and coronary artery disease.

Cardiomyopathy: Cardiomyopathy, also known as heart muscle disease, is basically a disease where the muscles of the heart get abnormally stiff, thick, or stretched. Genetic conditions, reactions to certain drugs and viral infections are believed to cause this disease, and the long-term survival of this disease is poor.

Cardiomyopathy is also linked to the development of other heart diseases like arrhythmias and heart failure.

Angina: Angina is just a fancy word for pain in the chest, sometimes also a squeezing sensation that is similar to indigestion. Angina is also a symptom of other heart conditions, and is common among a good percentage of individuals today.

Congenital Heart Disease: This disease is a simple term for a heart defect or abnormality that is present from birth. This may be caused while the fetus is still inside the uterus, and may occur due to exposure to certain chemicals, viruses, bacteria or use of certain medications.

Chapter 2: Treat Heart Disease- The Diet Way

Our diet plays an essential role in shaping our health and wellness, we all know that. Many of the foods that we eat today are nowhere near 'healthy,' which can be a great factor for concern. There are too many people who live on store-bought packaged foods and take-away meals from the roadside food joint, which is loaded with chemicals and preservatives, and sometimes prepared in unhygienic conditions. These foods have a good way of catching up to you later in life, and prolonged consumption of this kind of unhealthy food is linked to an increased risk of several heart diseases.

On the other hand, a healthy diet and lifestyle can cut down your risk of chronic health problems like diabetes, osteoporosis, high blood pressure, elevated cholesterol levels, obesity, stroke, heart attacks and other heart diseases as well.

While healthy eating habits in general, do have their own place of honor in preventing several heart diseases, the Mediterranean diet in particular, is thought to be one of the best diets that help individuals at a higher risk of suffering from different heart diseases.

Infact, the findings from a new study, published in the New England Journal of Medicine, revealed a 30 percent reduced risk of heart attacks, strokes and deaths from those who have similar diets to that of a Mediterranean diet, that is complete with fresh fruits and vegetables, olive oil, nuts, beans and fish.

This probably explains why people from the Mediterranean countries have a much lower risk of dying of heart and cardiovascular disease.

While there's practically no one-size-fits-all diet for those suffering from, or at a risk of heart disease, there are some foods and practical lifestyle tips that can help almost everyone out there keep their heart happy. **Below are some of the best tips and foods that can boost your heart health.**

Watch your portion size: Overeating is a strict no-no when it comes to switching to a heart-healthy diet. How much you eat also plays an important role- so make sure you wait for at least 10-15 minutes before going for second helpings whenever you eat.

Instead of eating a full meal three times a day, choose to break it down into smaller servings throughout the day- this prevents the digestive system from getting overloaded and also speeds up your metabolism. This is something most pro athletes and peak performers do as well. I made this change to my lifestyle several years ago and it is one of the best things I've ever done!

Go whole-grain: There is a good reason why Whole grains make it to the top of the list of foods to consider when it comes to improving your heart health. They are packed with the essential fiber and other heart-healthy nutrients that make them a must-have to add to your diet.

However, with the arrival of a number of new products in the market, claiming to be heart-healthy, you can get confused over which one really lives up to its name. Well, here I've put down some whole grain products you should definitely consider adding to your meals, and the ones you shouldn't.

Add these: Choose whole-wheat flour, whole-grain bread (preferably 100% whole-wheat or whole-grain), whole grains like brown rice, barley, buckwheat, high-fiber cereal, whole-grain pasta, oatmeal and flaxseed.

Skip these: Avoid packaged foods like white bread, doughnuts, white flour, refined flour, cakes, pies, granola bars, quick bread, biscuits, frozen waffles, muffins, corn bread, buttered popcorn and high-fat crackers.

Grab the fruits and veggies: This one's a no-brainer. Fresh fruits and vegetables are packed with essential micronutrients that help prevent cardiovascular diseases. They are low in calories and high in dietary fiber, which can help promote overall wellbeing.

The best way to get your daily requirement of heart-healthy vitamins and minerals is to keep raw fruits and vegetables in your kitchen or places where you'll see them (and probably eat them) often. Choose fresh fruits and veggies instead of cooked or canned ones that may contain preservatives and sodium. Avoid vegetables that come with creamy sauces and syrups, or frozen foods which have added sugar.

One of my favorite ways to get my daily dose of fruits and vegetables is by juicing and making smoothies. My two favorite products for doing this are: For Juicing: Breville Juice Fountain and for making smoothies: Nutri Bullet High Speed Blender.

Think low-fat: Let's face it, fatty foods are tempting and look more delicious than other foods; but here, we're specifically talking about low-fat protein sources. If you like to eat meat, try and choose lean meats like poultry, fish and seafood, and stick to egg whites and low-fat dairy products for your protein. Avoid processed and cured meats and try to choose skinless meats.

Another good idea is to add those meats that contain high levels of omega-3 fatty acids, such as fish and seafood, particularly mackerel, salmon and herring, to your diet. While choosing vegetarian proteins, stick to beans and lentils- they contain less fat and practically no cholesterol, which makes them the sure healthier choice over animal meats.

Resist the temptation to pick up hot dogs, sausages, bacon, fried meats, cold cuts, marbled meats and organ meats; your body will thank you for it later!

Skip the butter: Let's admit it, many people love those cheesy burgers and crisp fries; but experts believe that it's this very 'fat' that raises your risk of several cardiovascular health conditions to exorbitant levels. The saturated and trans fats, that can make up a large portion of what we eat, can increase blood cholesterol levels, and simultaneously raise the risk of coronary artery disease too! High blood cholesterol levels have also been linked to a higher risk of several other heart diseases including plaque build-up, heart attacks and stroke.

Thankfully, the American Heart Association has laid down a few guidelines for the ideal intake of different types of fats in the diet- saturated fats should make up less than 7 percent of your total calorie intake per day, trans fats should be responsible for less than 1 percent of the total calories you take in per day, and it is recommended that you should stick to less than 300 mg of cholesterol in your diet everyday.

This ideal ratio can be achieved by simply switching from butter, bacon fat, margarine, shortening, non-dairy creamer, cream sauce, lard, coconut oil, palm oil and cocoa butters to olive oil, canola oil and margarine's that are free from trans fats.

Cut down on the sodium: Higher sodium levels in the blood have been linked to an increased risk of high blood pressure and other cardiovascular diseases. The recommended daily intake for a healthy adult, according to the Department of Agriculture, is no more than 2300mg of sodium. For individuals who have been diagnosed with high blood pressure, chronic kidney disease or diabetes, 1500 mg per day should be the limit.

A simple and easy way to cut down on your sodium consumption would be to avoid packaged and processed foods- they contain higher levels of sodium than you might imagine. Instead, cook your meals yourself, with no salt, and then, right when you sit down to eat, sprinkle some salt over your food- that way, you'll be taking in a much lesser amount of sodium than you usually do. I have also recently switched out salt for seasoning on my foods with various herbs and spices. It is much healthier and I think it makes the food taste even better than salt would. Some herbs and spices you may want to try include: Garlic powder, Onion powder, Italian seasonings, Oregano leaves, Basil leaves, and a variety of other delicious and healthy herbs and spices.

It is also a good idea to avoid using soy sauce, ketchup, canned soups, canned beans, frozen dinners, tomato juice and other similar items to your food preparations.

Exercise: A healthy diet and moderate physical activity go hand-in-hand when it comes to getting heart healthy; and if you've been a couch potato for long, its time to get up and exercise.

I'll be focusing in detail about how exercise plays its own special role in boosting heart health in the 5th chapter. So stay tuned...

Chapter 3: The Medicinal Approach to Heart Diseases

Conventional medicines and drugs are the most popular treatment forms when it comes to dealing with heart diseases- and why not? Popping a pill is easier than anything else, right?

The downside, however, is that most of these medications and drugs carries with them a good number of side effects. However, here, I'll be explaining in general the different medications which you may be using (or can use) to help manage your heart problem.

Also, keep in mind that this book is for instructional purposes only-the common medications that I've listed below are just to educate you about how they work. It is of utmost importance to seek medical advice before starting with any of these drugs.

Aldosterone inhibitor: Aldosterone inhibitors help reduce swelling and build-up of water caused due to heart failure. They help the kidneys get rid of excess water and salts, and help maintain an optimum salt-water balance in the body. They also help protect the heart by blocking the production of a hormone named Aldosterone, which may cause salt and fluid build-up in the body.

Aldosterone inhibitors are frequently prescribed to individuals with severe heart failure.

ACE inhibitor: ACE inhibitors act by helping the arteries dilate (widen), which makes it easier for the blood to pass through them. They may also help to stop the harmful responses of the endocrine system that may occur due to heart failure.

Calcium-channel blockers: Calcium channel blockers work by altering the movement of calcium cells of the heart and blood vessels, which in turn causes an increased supply of oxygen and blood to the heart, improving its functioning. Calcium channel blockers are usually prescribed to individuals who suffer from high blood pressure and angina (chest pain). They may also prove to be an effective treatment against heart failure occurring as a result of high blood pressure.

Beta blockers: Beta blockers are substances that block the effects of the hormone adrenaline, improve the heart's ability to perform, and reduce the production of other harmful substances in the body which may affect heart health.

Cholesterol lowering drugs: As the name suggests, cholesterol lowering drugs are aimed at reducing the cholesterol levels in blood, bringing them down to safer levels and thereby cutting down the risk of build-up on the arterial walls, which may subsequently lead to an increased risk of heart attacks and stroke.

Vasodilators: Vasodilators are basically drugs that help control high blood pressure by relaxing the walls of the blood vessels, making the blood flow more easily through the vessels. They are generally used to treat heart failure, and are often prescribed to individuals who cannot take ACE inhibitors.

Diuretics: Generally prescribed as a drug for patients suffering from high blood pressure, diuretics are also known as water pills. They basically help the kidneys excrete excess water and salt from the tissues, and into the urine, which makes it easier for your heart to pump blood. They can also act as an effective treatment against conditions that worsen due to swelling and accumulation of water in the tissues of the body, including heart failure.

Be sure to contact your doctor for any professional medical advice you may need.

Chapter 4: Combat Heart Disease Naturally!

Looking for some natural ways to beat heart disease? Well, that's what this book is all about. Now that you've understood the basics of heart disease and how conventional medicine helps manage it, it's now time to discover the best natural treatments you can use to handle your heart condition or any potential future heart problems.

Here are some of the best tried and tested natural treatments in detail, and you can use them easily without much trouble at all. Best of all, since these therapies are natural, you can try them without any fear of very many side effects. However, make sure you seek professional medical advice before getting started with ANY of these therapies. Remember that most natural therapies and treatments are NOT a substitute for medical help- they are supposed to speed up your recovery, not work as the only treatment.

Acupressure: Acupressure and acupuncture- the two branches of traditional Chinese medicine, are among the most popular treatments used for heart diseases. While acupressure can be done by almost anyone, acupuncture therapy may require the assistance of a qualified practitioner. But don't worry, both of them work on the same principle, and use the same approach to help strengthen your heart and help you lead a healthy, active life.

Acupressure and acupuncture work by stimulating certain points on the body, which trigger healing reactions in the body. It is also believed that most of the diseases occurring in the body, including heart disease, happen due to an imbalance in the energy travelling through the body. By stimulating certain points on the body using the fingers (in acupressure) or needles (in acupuncture), the energy blockages can be removed, and the body enters a state of well being.

Practicing acupressure yourself isn't difficult- you can do it even if you have no prior experience. However, it is important to have a talk with your general practitioner before starting out with acupressure, just to make sure you're free from any potential health risks.

Here I've listed down a few acupressure points- you can stimulate them by applying pressure using your fingers.

Point #1: Mind Door

This point is believed to be the source point of the heart. You can locate this point on the palm side of your hand on the wrist crease below your tiny finger. A good trick to find the correct point is to gently press the area around the given location, and find the region that feels most sensitive and tender. Most of the time, these points on the body, corresponding to the different body regions, are tender and sensitive if they have some problem, which makes it easy to locate them.

Apply pressure on this point (on both the hands), by holding for 10 seconds, and then releasing for 2 seconds. Do this for 2-3 minutes on each hand. It is recommended to do this regularly as it is believed to send nourishment to the heart and prevent many heart diseases.

Point #2: Inner Gate

This point is also known as the heart protector. Stimulating this point regularly can strengthen your heart and relive pain and discomfort in the chest. This point can be found near your wrist on the palm side, and two thumb widths above the crease of the wrist, in the center of the palm.

Make sure you apply pressure on both the hands. Ideally, the pressure shouldn't be too light, or too strong- it should be firm and gentle. Hold for 10 seconds and then release for 2 seconds.

You can also check out these great YouTube videos to understand other acupressure points that help you to improve your heart health.

Stop Chest Pain Fast with Massage & Acupressure by VitalityMassage

Acupressure Healing Point for the Heart by Dr. Larry Caldwell

Naturopathy: Naturopathy is yet another popular form of alternative medicine which is believed to have helped millions of individuals suffering from heart disease deal with their condition in a better, more effective way.

Naturopathic approaches include incorporating simple diet and lifestyle changes to speed up healing and recovery. It also involves the use of effective preventive measures to help prevent the disease from affecting the individual. Multivitamin and mineral supplements are often used as a part of naturopathic treatments to help boost organ health and improve body function.

In naturopathy, processed and packaged food consumption is discouraged, and raw foods are preferred. Sometimes, a naturopath may also ask you to follow a particular diet pertaining to your health condition, such as a Mediterranean diet, which is commonly used for individuals who suffer from heart disease. Yet another important part of a naturopathic treatment for heart disease is the use of special packs and baths, which are believed to have healing properties and benefits for the body, particularly the heart.

Lastly, naturopathic medicine also stresses the importance of positive thinking as a part of well being and health, which seems pretty true, as a lot of the health problems people suffer from today are, in one way or the other, linked to stress, depression, anxiety and other psychological problems. For great strategies to improve your mood, be sure to check out my E-Book: Laughter Therapy.

Herbal medicine: Herbal medicine has been an essential part of many natural healing therapies, and that's pretty obvious. Using botanical and herbal extracts, a good state of health can be achieved pretty easily if everything is done correctly. The best benefit of using herbal medicine to manage your heart condition is that these herbs carry minimum or no side effects associated with their use, as opposed to other medications and drugs.

Here are some of the best herbs and plants that can be good for heart problems.

Garlic: Garlic is the best known botanical that has been known for its importance in boosting heart heath. Just a single clove of garlic a day has the power to regulate cholesterol levels in blood, and bring blood pressure back to normal in most people.

Green tea: Green tea is packed with antioxidants that improve heart health, fight free radicals and boost overall performance. It is also believed that drinking green tea can improve blood vessel function.

Oregano: Oregano is a rich natural source of antioxidants and vitamin C, which helps fight free radicals and prevent a number of heart diseases and even cancer.

Fenugreek: Fenugreek seeds are known for their efficacy in improving digestive health, but a few studies suggest that regular consumption of these seeds may boost heart health as well. These seeds are amazingly effective in shrinking plaque deposits and decreasing high blood cholesterol levels.

Grapes: Grapes are thought to contain important phytomedicinal compounds that protect the cardiovascular system from damage and protect it against free radical damage.

Motherwort: Simply put, motherwort is not a simple herb- it's a heart tonic. The substances found in motherwort are believed to slow down a rapid heart rate, strengthen the heart and reduce platelet accumulation. Some research also suggests that motherwort may help reduce blood cholesterol.

Cayenne pepper: Used as a seasoning for many dishes and foods, cayenne pepper is blessed with many cholesterol-lowering properties, which makes it a must have for those suffering from heart conditions. Cayenne pepper is also believed to contain antioxidants that protect the heart from free radical damage.

Dark chocolate: This one's probably the best- dark chocolate contains many essential antioxidants that prevent heart attacks, stroke and other cardiovascular events. It also contains a compound known as flavonols, which reduces cell damage occurring in heart disease.

Olive oil: Olive oil possesses some of the best antioxidant and heart-protecting compounds, which make it the number one natural treatment against several heart conditions. Regular consumption of olive oil is believed to cut down the risk of stroke and coronary artery disease.

Before using any herbal medicine, make sure you seek the advice of your doctor-though most herbs do not have any side effects; they may have certain drug interactions you may not know about. Speak to your healthcare provider about the safety of taking herbs for your heart health, and be sure to check and rule out any allergic reactions you may have.

Yoga: There's a reason why yoga is so popular- it has been tried and tested, and millions of people from around the world have experienced the benefits of trying yoga exercises to deal with their heart problems and other health concerns.

Basically, yoga breathing exercises and body positions work by improving the flow of oxygen into the blood, purifying it, and thereby strengthening the organs of the body, including the heart. Most yoga positions also include poses that stimulate the release of toxins from the body, which could potentially have caused heart problems, and yoga is great for improving the overall health of the body.

It is also believed that some yoga practices can boost the natural healing energies of the body, and thereby prevent many other diseases too.

Here are some effective yoga positions that could help you to improve your heart health, and also help you to lead a more energetic, and healthy life.

Natrajasana: The natrajasana is also known as the dancing Shiva pose, and is best for providing strength to the heart and relieving stress.

This may not be achievable for everyone, but there are many health benefits for trying too. Start by standing straight, and as you breathe in, move your right hand and leg backwards, and stretch them till they meet each other on the back side of your body. Hold this pose till you can, and then breathe out as you slowly release the pose. To see exactly how this is done check out this YouTube video by Shilpa's Yoga : Yoga for Hip, Thighs & Chest - Natrajasana.

Ardhachandrasana: This position is believed to help strengthen the heart and chest muscles, and is also known as the crescent pose.

Stand with your feet a little apart, and place your hands on your waist. Now, inhale slowly and tilt your head upwards slightly, causing your chest to expand, and then come back to the normal position as you exhale.

Tadasana: Also known as the palm tree pose, this yoga position is pretty simple, and holds many benefits for the heart. It is known to help massage the internal organs of the body, particularly the chest region, and improve heart strength.

Stand up straight on your toes, and your hands high up in the air, palms facing each other as you inhale. Hold this pose for a couple of seconds and then exhale, coming back to the ground. Perform this cycle for at least 10 times a day for maximum benefits.

You can also check out these great videos on YouTube, which show you how to perform simple yoga poses that improve heart health.

4 Poses to Cure Heart Diseases by vimalvyas

Yoga Exercise to Cure Heart Disease by Yoga

Yoga For A Healthy Heart by mydailyyoga

You can also check out books and dvd's that emphasize yoga to improve general health and in particular heart health. If you don't find the time to practice yoga daily, make sure you take deep, long breaths whenever you can, throughout the day- this will improve the flow of oxygen into your body and strengthen your heart muscles, making you less susceptible to heart disorders.

Psychological therapies: Just like the food we take, our mindset and belief also plays an important role in determining our health. This is probably why psychological therapies prove to be quite helpful in preventing and managing heart diseases.

Here are some creative visualization techniques that may help you. Set out 10 minutes from your day for this simple exercise, preferably, right after you wake up in the morning. Start by lying down in a comfortable position. Take slow, deep breaths and relax your mind as much as possible. Now imagine yourself as a super powerful energetic being that is radiating light from your chest, right where your heart is. Visualize yourself gliding through the day's activity with ease and perfection, imagine your heart getting better and stronger, with every breath imagine healing waves of pure energy all around your heart.

Do this exercise as often as you like, but preferably at least once a day. This exercise can help your mind and your body get on the same spiritual level, which can be very beneficial to your overall health.

Other therapies: Under alternative and natural medicine, you'll find many other therapies that may help you manage your heart condition better. Here I've listed down some of the best therapies you can try.

- Aura healing: Aura healing is a unique alternative therapy, which helps the practitioner determine exactly where the health problem lies, and then attempts to help with the problem in a spiritual way. Many people are extremely fond of this type of therapy, and others say that it does not work.

- Pet therapy: This is a relatively new therapy, but has been found to be very effective in the treatment of stress and heart disease. Spending some time with your pet causes your body to release healing hormones, which improves your overall health.

- Laughter therapy: This therapy works on the same basis as pet therapy, and is quite popular nowadays, especially as an anger management therapy. It encourages the mind to feel happy and light, releases stress and improves heart health and promotes overall well-being. If you would like to know more about Laughter Therapy feel free to get one of my bestselling books: Laughter Therapy.

- Color therapy: Color therapy works on the belief that different colors have an impact on your health, and can improve or worsen your condition.

- Aromatherapy: Aromatherapy uses the power of different fragrances, essential oils, and essences to accelerate internal healing and bring about a variety of different mental states, depending on which fragrance, essential oil, or essence you are using. Here is a great diffuser you can get on Amazon: Aromatherapy essential oil diffuser. Some of my favorite essential oils to use are: Peppermint, Verbena, Cinnamon, and Rosemary.

- Reiki: Reiki healing therapy uses the healing energies from the practitioner to the patient, which is said to accelerate healing. Here is a YouTube video by Healing Light Reiki showing it in use: Reiki Treatment Session.

- Crystal therapy: Crystal therapy makes use of the power of crystals to spread positive, healing energies around you, which is said to bring about health and wellness. Here is a video on YouTube about Crystal Therapy by CrystalAgeTV: How To Use Crystals In Healing.

- Ayurveda: Ayurveda is yet another effective age-old therapy that may help you manage your heart disease better. Here is a nice video on YouTube by TKG2288 that goes into more detail: The Secret World of Wellness Ayurveda Ancient India.

- Massage therapy: Massage therapy has tremendous benefits for the body and the mind, and my personal favorite. The health benefits of a full body massage done by a professional are legendary.

Chapter 5: Sweat it Out- How Exercise Helps

Lack of exercise is one of the major factors that can raise the risk of cardiovascular diseases; fortunately, it's something you can do something about. If you've been leading a sedentary lifestyle with minimal physical activity, take charge of your life and start exercising now.

Aerobic exercises, in particular, hold many health benefits when it comes to the heart- practicing aerobic exercises daily can-

- Increase your endurance.
- Lower high blood pressure levels.
- Improve blood circulation and oxygenate the body.
- Improve heart health.
- Strengthen the heart and the cardiovascular system.
- Strengthen the bones.
- Boost muscle and joint health.
- Give you an energy boost that keeps you fit and active throughout the day.
- Prevents fatigue and weakness.
- Improves sleep cycles and prevents sleep disorders.
- Helps improve your balance and joint flexibility.
- Prevents occurrence of psychological disorders like depression, stress, anxiety, nervousness and low self esteem.
- Keeps you more relaxed and calm.
- Improves metabolism and prevents obesity.
- Keeps you looking more fit and healthy.

Researchers believe that just 30 minutes of moderate physical activity, done 3 times a week, can cut down your risk of developing heart disease by 20 to 60 percent!

It is speculated that this direct link between exercise and a lower risk of heart disease may be due to the fact that exercising reduces blood pressure, which is a major risk factor that contributes to the development of other heart conditions. Yet another study has revealed how exercising can cause the body to transport a greater number of stem cells to the heart, which in turn, can possibly repair damaged heart cells, naturally promoting the healing process.

What's more, regular exercise is known to reduce triglyceride and cholesterol levels, which when deposited onto the arteries, can cause blood pressure problems and restricted blood flow.

Heart-Healthy Exercise Guide: It seems I've convinced you enough; and now it's time to move on and explore some great exercise tips and tricks that can help improve your heart's health.

First and foremost, it's important to take some time out from your day and dedicate it to exercise- preferably 30 minutes. It could also be a good idea to consult your doctor before starting any high-strain resistance exercises like weight training or high strain cardiovascular exercise like running.

Ideally, your exercise routine should begin with a warm-up, which ensures that your body is in the exercise mode, has a far less chance of injury, and will allow it to perform better during your exercise routine. Next comes the conditioning phase, where the exercise moves on to its full-effect- be sure to monitor your heart rate here, especially if your doctor suggests that you do so. The final phase of the exercise should be a cool-down phase, where you bring your body to rest and allow it to recover from the conditioning phase. Walking is one of the best cool-down techniques.

Warm-up shouldn't take more than 10-15 minutes of your workout session, and be sure you incorporate stretching and motion exercises to prevent muscle soreness and increase flexibility. On a similar note, the cool-down session should include stretching exercises and performing the same exercise that you were just doing in the conditioning phase, only at a lighter level, which can help your heart rate and blood pressure go back to normal.

To make things even easier, I've put down some simple exercises you can try to boost your heart health.

Swimming: Swimming is an all-around great exercise. Swimming can be a good way to burn some calories, get fit and boost your heart health at the same time. Try swimming laps or participate in a water fitness class- they improve your heart health and boost muscle strength too! Also, swimming is a good exercise alternative for those who suffer from joint problems like rheumatism and arthritis. One of the huge advantages of swimming is not only increased strength, but the chances of you getting injured during a workout are far lower than that of other exercises.

Walking: Walking is the simplest and easiest way to get fit and active- whether you do it on the road, in the fresh air, or in a gym on the treadmill, it is the most natural way to improve your heart's function. Make sure you achieve a moderate intensity while walking- neither too fast, nor too slow. This is another of my favorite exercises. I see great results, it's easy to get myself motivated to go outside and walk in nature, and just like swimming, the chances of you getting injured while walking are greatly reduced compared to other exercises.

Cycling: Cycling is yet another physical activity that's great for the heart, yet easy on your knees and other joints. This low-impact exercise can be coupled with some other tasks, like getting to the supermarket to buy some food, or a short bike trip with friends. Cycling is also believed to help tone your lower body and strengthen your muscles, improving resistance.

Running: If you're in a mood to get a bit more active, running could be the best for both- you and your heart. Running is more challenging than walking, and is a good way to burn a lot of calories in a short period of time. If you're a new to running, start out with some stretching exercises, then move on to a brisk walk for your warm up, and then increase your pace after 5-10 minutes. Make sure you slow down your pace for 1-2 minutes for every 5 minutes of running, so that you don't put an extra strain on your heart.

Internal training: If regular running and walking bores you to the core, interval training could be an interesting exercise routine to try out. Just add a couple of minutes of strength training or some high intensity training exercises to every 3 minutes of cardio. Alternatively, you could also choose 5 different high intensity exercises and do 1 set of each, and then move on to moderate exercise- this will help keep your heart rate up and increase your endurance, keeping you motivated.

Conclusion

I hope this book was able to help you give you a fresh insight about your heart condition, and that you now know some great strategies and techniques to try and keep your heart healthy and strong! Just a few simple lifestyle changes can make a huge difference. Now that you know how our lifestyle choices can affect 90% of our health outcomes, it's time to buckle up and make healthier lifestyle choices, for a better tomorrow.

The next step is to take charge of your health- make a determined decision to take steps into improving your heart health. Remember that taking baby steps counts too! Just a little effort, some small lifestyle and food changes, and a positive outlook on life is all you need to boost your health and get your heart happy!

Never underestimate the power of food- just choosing the right foods (like the ones I've listed in this book), and exercising could bring you many benefits. So what are you waiting for? Get up and start your journey towards a better life and a stronger and healthier heart.

Finally, if you discovered at least one thing that has helped you or that you think would be beneficial to someone else, be sure to take a few seconds to easily post a quick positive review. As an author, your positive feedback is desperately needed. Your highly valuable five star reviews are like a river of golden joy flowing through a sunny forest of mighty trees and beautiful flowers! *To do your good deed in making the world a better place by helping others with your valuable insight, just leave a nice review.*

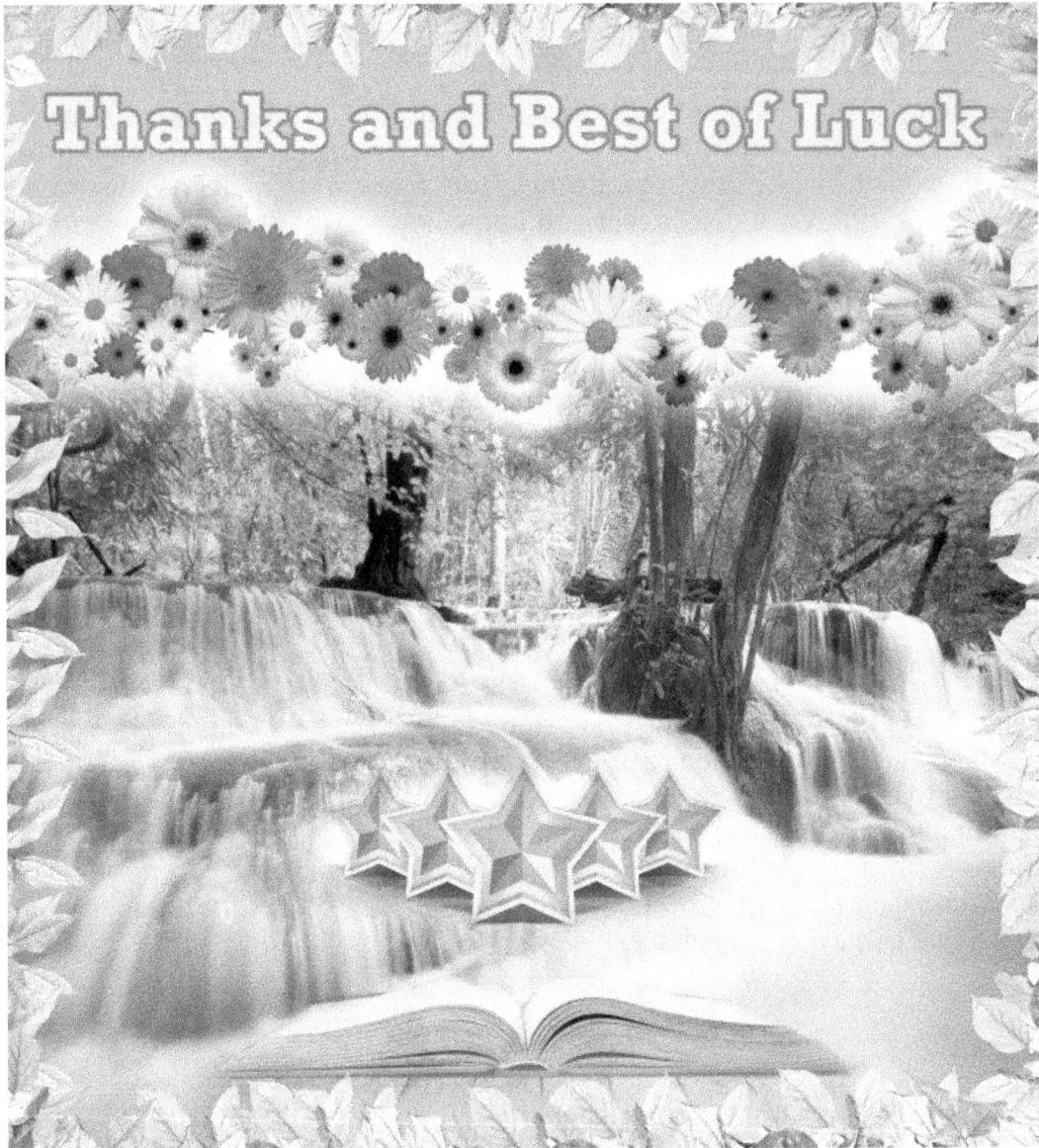

Thanks and Best of Luck

My Other Books and Audio Books
www.AcesEbooks.com

Health Books

ULTIMATE HEALTH SECRETS

HEALTH

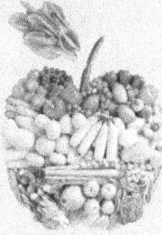

Strategies For Dieting, Eating Healthy, Exercising, Losing Weight, The Mediterranean Diet, Strength Training, And All About Vitamins, Minerals, And Supplements

Ace McCloud

ENERGY
ULTIMATE ENERGY

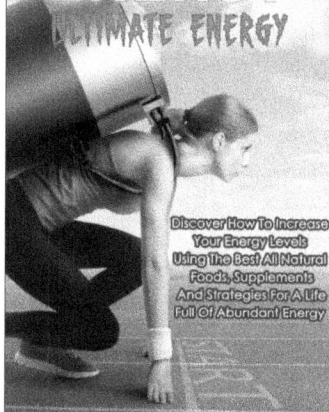

Discover How To Increase Your Energy Levels Using The Best All Natural Foods, Supplements And Strategies For A Life Full Of Abundant Energy

Ace McCloud

RECIPE BOOK

The Best Food Recipes That Are Delicious, Healthy, Great For Energy And Easy To Make

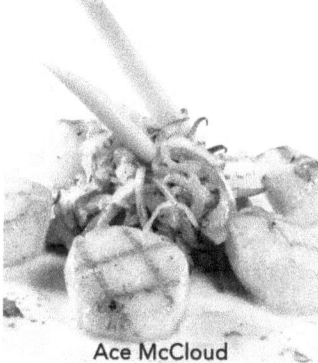

Ace McCloud

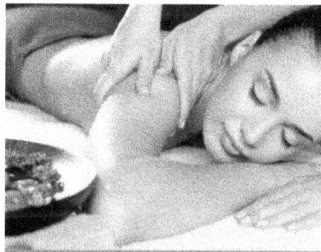

MASSAGE THERAPY

TRIGGER POINT THERAPY
ACUPRESSURE THERAPY
Learn The Best Techniques For Optimum Pain Relief And Relaxation

Ace McCloud

LOSE WEIGHT

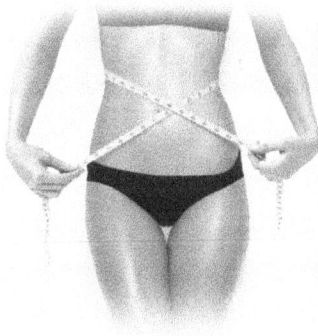

THE TOP 100 BEST WAYS TO LOSE WEIGHT QUICKLY AND HEALTHILY

Ace McCloud

FATIGUE
OVERCOME CHRONIC FATIGUE

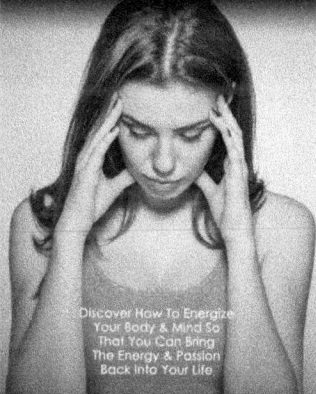

Discover How To Energize Your Body & Mind So That You Can Bring The Energy & Passion Back Into Your Life

Ace McCloud

Peak Performance Books

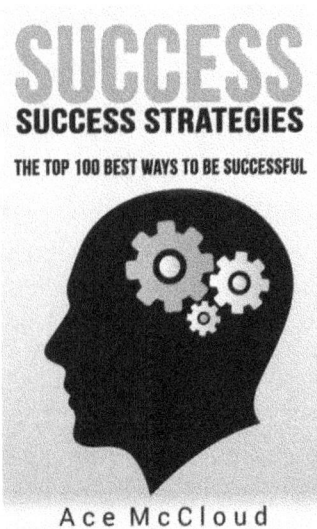

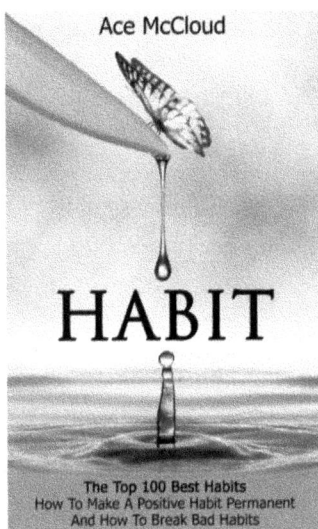

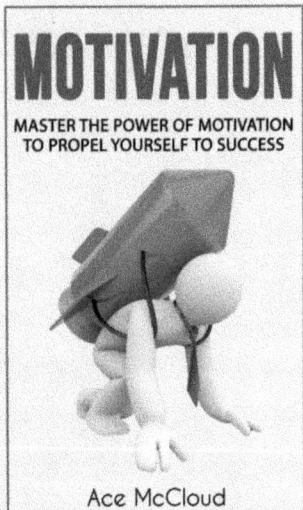

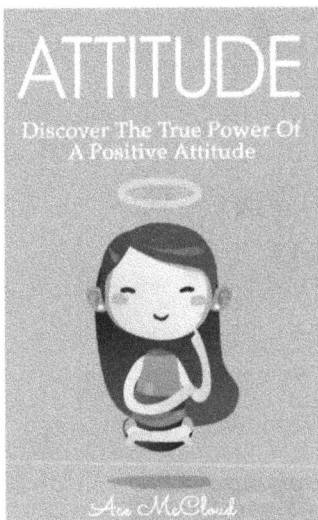

SUCCESS
SUCCESS STRATEGIES
THE TOP 100 BEST WAYS TO BE SUCCESSFUL
Ace McCloud

Ace McCloud
HABIT
The Top 100 Best Habits
How To Make A Positive Habit Permanent
And How To Break Bad Habits

MOTIVATION
MASTER THE POWER OF MOTIVATION
TO PROPEL YOURSELF TO SUCCESS
Ace McCloud

ATTITUDE
Discover The True Power Of
A Positive Attitude
Ace McCloud

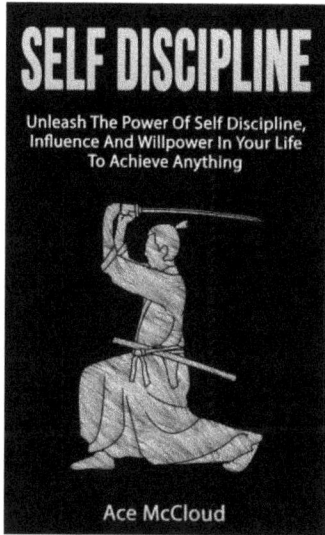

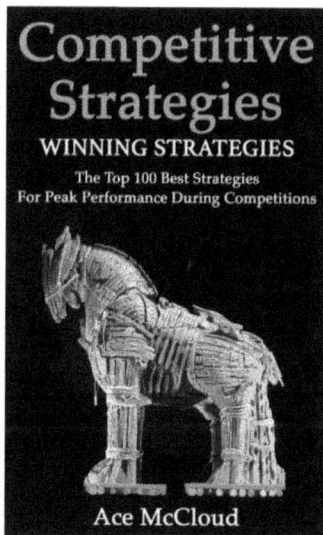

Be sure to check out my audio books as well!

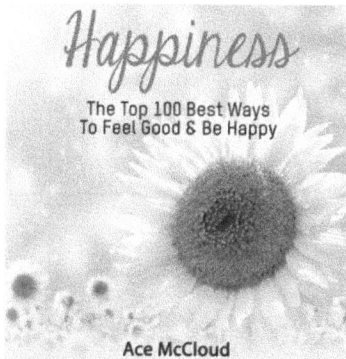

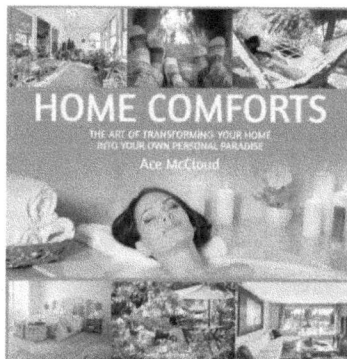

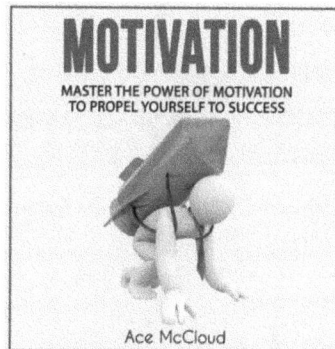

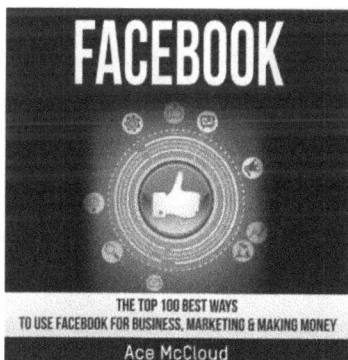

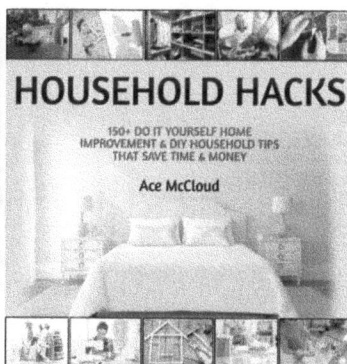

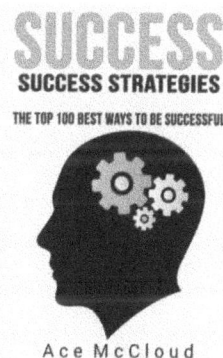

Check out my website at: **www.AcesEbooks.com** for a complete list of all of my books and high quality audio books. I enjoy bringing you the best knowledge in the world and wish you the best in using this information to make your journey through life better and more enjoyable! **Best of luck to you!**